The Test of Non-Duality

Yogic Kriya for Intense Spiritual Purification
Transcending the Dark Night of Soul

Sukhendu Mandal, PhD.

BALBOA.PRESS
A DIVISION OF HAY HOUSE

Balboa Press books may be ordered through booksellers or by contacting:

Balboa Press
A Division of Hay House
1663 Liberty Drive
Bloomington, IN 47403
www.balboapress.com
844-682-1282

Because of the dynamic nature of the Internet, any web addresses or links contained in this book may have changed since publication and may no longer be valid. The views expressed in this work are solely those of the author and do not necessarily reflect the views of the publisher, and the publisher hereby disclaims any responsibility for them.

The author of this book does not dispense medical advice or prescribe the use of any technique as a form of treatment for physical, emotional, or medical problems without the advice of a physician, either directly or indirectly. The intent of the author is only to offer information of a general nature to help you in your quest for emotional and spiritual well-being. In the event you use any of the information in this book for yourself, which is your constitutional right, the author and the publisher assume no responsibility for your actions.

Any people depicted in stock imagery provided by Getty Images are models, and such images are being used for illustrative purposes only. Certain stock imagery © Getty Images.

Interior Image Credit: Sukhendu Mandal

Print information available on the last page.

ISBN: 979-8-7652-3824-0 (sc)
ISBN: 979-8-7652-3825-7 (e)

Balboa Press rev. date: 01/23/2023

Disclaimer

All the information shared in this book is for educational purposes. Yoga practice in any form must be part of a daily healthy routine. This information must not be perceived as a quick fix for personal problems and may not serve the purpose. Under no situation, this information be applied to medical diagnosis or used as an alternative to medical treatment. The sole purpose of yogic practice is to bring consciousness to different aspects of the self.

Every individual responds differently to this type of work, and the person will be solely responsible for all the outcomes. The author does not take the responsibility for any direct or indirect effects that the reader/user may experience. The information may or may not align with every reader's personal and cultural beliefs. Reader's discretion is advised.

Contents

Keywords

Mind/Personality/ID: These terms are used interchangeably and designates the functioning program in a person

Non-Duality: A spiritual philosophy that perceives everything as one and has no opposites like good or evil

Initiation: A spiritual process of activation

Spiritual discipline: Any form of spiritual practice

Self realization: Becoming fully aware of how one functions (perceives, receives, and acts)

Self Actualization: A term used similarly to Realization but refers more as creating the realized self

Spiritual energy: A medium or form named as energy that could be transferred from spiritual teachers (This does not have existence as energy in physics)

Kundalini: The spiritual energy contained in the spine of an individual generally locked at root

Initiate: A spiritual practitioner aimed to attain higher consciousness

Mudra: Hand position in yoga

Introduction

Test of Non-Duality is the third book in the Beyond Placebo project. It is almost a decade now since the idea of studying, understanding, and sharing Indian yogic systems initiated. Over the years, this project met with, learned from, and trained many yogis and spiritual seekers worldwide. The project has evolved into a vast resource of knowledge and spiritual consciousness that has been shared with the book series. Thousands of people have read and applied these simplified techniques to heal different aspects of their life. It is said these concepts are beyond time and have amplified the spiritual transition this world is going through.

With this title, the author shares yet another gem in the path of spiritual transformation, rarely discussed among seekers and practitioners. Only those in the advanced states of spiritual consciousness are aware of these situations that seekers struggle with in their path. This book was inspired by interaction with advanced yogis and healers struggling with all types of spiritual and practical problems. It takes years before they realize the darkness was a result of their own spiritual work. This darkness born out of spiritual light could not be transcended with any form of spiritual and energy work, and created the spiritual trap.

Keeping in mind the advanced seekers, healers, and spiritual teachers, this book shares an intensive process of spiritual purification that transcends all distortions of duality. Test of Non-duality is the heightened state where the seeker has the opportunity to transcend the hidden ignorance and perfectly align with the consciousness of freedom.

This special spiritual discipline has connections with ancient Indian yogic systems and shared accordingly. It was one of the author's most intense spiritual experiences in all these years. The process not only helps spiritual seekers learn from their own mistakes but also realize the ignorance spiritual practice has been hiding all along.

Connecting the dots

THIS BOOK IS THE MOST extended project among the four in this series. The publishing contract is almost two years old now. For some reason, this kept on being delayed. I was a naïve author and equally lazy; then, the computer and laptop crashed simultaneously, followed by the pandemic situation. There is another reason for not being able to fulfill the publishing contract. It is the conscious energy field of this yogic knowledge. Every time I tried to sit and write on this project, it would put me into an energetic whirlpool, and the energies would spin at full swing, making my thoughts cloudy. All I could do at this point was fall asleep.

Recently, I shifted to Chandigarh to apply Post Doctoral fellowship in Mind-Body intervention. I had to visit the university to interact with other scholars and guides. This afternoon I met a few scholars in the field of Yoga and Consciousness research. One of them recently submitted his thesis on Kriya yog. That evening passed in scholarly discussions and I had the chance to visit one of the sacred sites in this city.

I acknowledged to the scholar that I had found the first chapter of my book, which means the project is ready for publication.

I remember what was to be the initiation point of this project. That lucid experience:

*The name, '**Maha Avtaar Babaji**' and that intense field of energy.*

A Dream

I WAS NEVER A DEDICATED writer. I have the patterns of volcano; years of silence and then a major eruption. At times, I would wake up at night and write an entire chapter. And then obsess for the whole year to write another one. Sometimes, I entirely dream a chapter theme because I was so grossly engaged in the writing for days. It is said that dreams reveal insights from our greatest wisdom. This was one of the most meaningful dream during the writing process. It is the most refined expression of my inner thoughts, that otherwise might not find a structure. Understanding the dream itself would have been the completion of the Test.

It was a place I lived during my childhood days. I walked out of my house and meet people around the place. Everyone had problems in their lives. I happen to be the one helping them all through. The types of problems were not shown in dream but it seems like a dark fog around the people. As a problem solver, I was interacting with people and clearing the dark fog. After interaction with multiple people, there was a view that the darkness cleared but some of the dark spills began to grow and spread like slime. The spills joined together forming a darker smog. This was the problem I ended up being stuck. I could not solve it with my tools.

Some way I was searching for help and wished for higher support. And then two men appeared. One of them was a Kung fu master while the other has beards that gives a sense of Lion Face or Monkey King. Their appearance itself was clearing the space. When they participated in destroying the dark slime it disappeared without any trace. Their ability to solve problems was fierce and it did not create any form of accumulations.

I was fully awake by now, smiling at the non-sense dream, at the same time, savoring the answer.

Soul in crisis

IT WAS A LONG-TERM SICKNESS that had the effect of disconnecting me from everything. I had the experience of reviewing everything in life and integrating the lessons with peak intensity. Not an easy phase, though; it has passed. By the time I could collect myself and take charge of my studies, it was probably gone. There was hardly any connection point for me. This was a one-way path.

Yoga practice

I was in a long-term practice in a system of Kundalini yoga. A form of lotus posture that instils compassion and focuses on chanting meditation. This early form of teaching in Indian Yoga did not go with any spiritual activation. The practitioner is supposed to figure out everything in the process. But it rarely works when one does not know what to expect in the process. Moreover, the teachings came with multiple distorted stories and beliefs from the teacher.

It is 16 years now, with a term of dedicated practice following some gaps. The discipline was to be of 14 years to complete the entire process. The problem was that the teaching missed a large part of the road map.

This sickness left me with a broken path to what was soon to be a new road map.

The Calling

The first time I encountered this name was during a tour. The second time was when I opened a book purchased from a second hand book market in Kolkata. The page I read had a mystical encounter with

Maha Avataar Babaji. The third time was a picture sent by a friend from an old temple with a picture of a Yogi named Maha Avatar Babaji. All this synchronicities in a short time when this book idea has shown its first glimpse.

The path of Purification

A major purging has already passed my life in the past 2 years. Now I had the choice to step out of the toxic cycle. It would mean leaving behind everything. It is about 16 years of practice without a roadmap. Finally, it is time to reach the consciousness that would create the path ahead. It is time I realize that I am the Source of my Yogic Path; I am the One I seek.

The rebirth process

That was the very first introduction of the Beyond Placebo project to the public. The seminars began in Bangalore at a place offered by one of my friends. The workshop was repeated for those who missed the weekend class. This time it was at my friend's house, who teaches various healing modalities. The morning half was her shamanic journey class, and the next half was for me. I reached her place an hour or two earlier and joined the Shamanic journey class. This is not something I have ever heard about.

After the drumming session, everyone shared their journey experiences. And what showed up for me was interpreted.

"You have gone through a rebirth," the Shamanic lady said.

Choose Integrated Path

KNOWING WHERE YOU STAND AND the direction you are headed before choosing this path is essential. There are no higher or lower levels in consciousness; all is One. Perceiving something as higher and the self as lower creates a meta of self-rejection and creates a disconnect with the Self. The fragmentation later shows up as magical thinking and dysfunctional behaviors. As the spiritual circuits begin to activate, a practitioner will start the journey of mystical experiences. Though they may seem extraordinary events, the experiences are based on subtle beliefs and perceptions. A large part of spiritual experiences is structured from the information one picks during early practices. The human mind uses this information as a landmark of spiritual progress. But the problem is that, all of it is still created in mind.

You are, and continue to be, the Creator of your Experiences.

When receiving initiation from a Guru, most initiates have mystical experiences and visions. It is part of an imprint from the guru and may have nothing to do with a higher reality. Not realizing this, people tend to lose connection with reality and start serving a projected dream.

Any practice that does not serve growth in your personal and practical life is dysfunctional. In a way, it is not for you. Some higher philosophies developed in the Himalayas serve better only in the Himalayas!

Learn, apply, and reject what does not serve your growth. Simple!

Beyond Placebo project has witnessed hundreds of mystical experiences in people around the country and readers worldwide. It is quite possible to induce spiritual experiences in self or in others. Suppose the experiences are inducible and are created in mind. In that case, all these mystical teachings and the search for the ultimate end up being an illusion. Is there any outcome to it? Soul, liberation, divine, truth, etc., all of it will seem to be a part of projected metaphors.

This knowledge is shared upfront before you begin the path. It will be an imaginably painful realization after decades spent in practice. The ultimate goal of any practice must be living with gentleness, joy, and openness to learning. Gentle self-discipline is enough to become a Master.

An integrated path is possible when one realizes the ultimate reality is practical and participates in practice with total acceptance of life. Such practitioners are less likely to have other dimensional experiences but live a vibrant and balanced life. On the other hand, unhappy people with rejection towards life seek higher worlds and end up with fragmented spiritual experiences. This is where all the spiritual drama begins. The play is not fruitful at all.

Strict discipline for 21 days

Unlike the first two books, this book will be different, and a rather serious tone will follow throughout. There is a specific reason for this. It is one of those works from Indian Yogic systems that needs intensive self-discipline and inner cultivation. It is like the early phase of creation and restructuring of the inner values. Lack of discernment and indiscipline might cause a significant distortion in the entire process of Self Realization. It is advisable not to step in the process unless one has decided the path of strict discipline and inner cultivation for the period needed in this practice.

This book was inspired by and partly written in 2017. The book's main content was developed in early 2018 seminars in Bangalore and

Mumbai. The concept has received some inspiration from Banaras as well. The core process took longer to refine than I thought, and it happened to be one of the most intense spiritual techniques ever written with this project.

This is also not one of those works that could be learned, mastered, and re-sold. While there is no judgment over the new-age spirituality marketing process, this does not go that way. The process follows the concept of the age-old yogic system whereby there are three levels of learning. In Japanese terms, it is called 'SHU-HA-RI'. The first would be learning and practicing as it is taught. The second is to practice through the challenges that appear. The last is transforming into an entirely new set of principles more suited to the practitioner. At this stage, the practitioner becomes one with the process and is ready to become a teacher. This book, with 21 days of practice, follows all three levels of spiritual transformation. The 21st day is the second most intense experience after the first. It is where the sacred geometries spread in the entire body activating all levels of the spiritual field.

The second cycle of 21 days allows the flow of awareness to new levels. After 42 days, a practitioner may stop and participate only when there is a desire to connect.

Free from Distortions

This system of practice is kept neutral and free from spiritual distortions. During the early part of writing and interaction with a population of advanced yogis, healers, and coaches, it was realized that a large amount of spiritual teachings has distorted values. This would show up as life problems in the long run. The entire issue was a wrong set of values in practice that would misalign the practitioner's mindset. The result was problems in life that are attributed to negative karma or negative energy. The practitioner has no direct way to identify and correct the issues because the mind only perceives the projection, not the reel in play.

Keep it Clean

As a practitioner, it is entirely up to you to decide the path and the outcome. It is often advised not to share your yogic practice concepts, goals, or experiences with anyone. There are multiple reasons for it. The most important reason is to keep it clear of negative thoughts and beliefs. It is usual for others to make abrupt comments over things they do not understand. This creates a subconscious response for the practitioner, which affects the practice outcome.

Stay safe from Manipulation

Even well-disciplined yogis are not safe from manipulation. The fastest, most effective method of manipulation people use is generally profoundly effective, and there is no firewall against it.

It is called 'Change the Definition'. The moment someone puts a different definition to what you have been aligned with for so long, it would create a cascade of responses in the entire subconscious. If the redefinition is a negative one, there is a quick negative response. This response again enforces the new definition. While in the first place, You have been manipulated.

This concept showed up while writing the part about narcissistic and psychopathic abuse. Toxic, manipulative people use unhealthy redefining tricks.

This day, healers and coaches also use manipulation to market their modality. This is a highly effective tool in grabbing clients from another modality. The end result is the client gets programmed for a negative response and unnecessarily suffers. This is the reason the current spiritual market has so many people experiencing negative energy, ghosts, aliens, and other fragmented aspects. Because of the experience, they are less likely to realize it was their inner response created due to a misaligned piece of information.

For this reason, most of my book has terminologies that are least related to old teachings. It would take just another author to say that they are a master in that 'Technique' and become an authentic point of manipulation to the readers.

Concerning this book and the yogic practice, make it clear. The technique is not from someone else, related to any mythology or religion, and no one in the upcoming time would be a master of this.

As a practitioner, you are the sole authentic person to decide and walk your path. This book is the well structured map to create and design the path.

One Discipline

The practice of this system follows one discipline rule. There are no harsh ways of self-control or any form of intense physical or mental work. The rule is to stay true and practice only one mudra during the entire cycle of purification for 21 days. The disciplining must be slow and consistent and allow the flow of grace. Practitioners are suggested not to combine different modalities to seek and explore other layers of experiences. This one practice is enough to allow access to all needed levels.

This practice is not for people with any form of addictions, chronic mental and emotional problems, or unhealthy sexual behaviors. Non-vegetarian food and alcohol are strictly prohibited. Though the participating groups have been liberal with non-vegetarian food, alcohol in any volume has put people totally off balance.

Then, what is not allowed is playing with the activation process or manipulating it. It is understandable that new healers and coaches like learning things and teaching others; it is advisable that you be a student and mature up to be a teacher. The transformation process is relatively smooth and graceful than recovering from fragmentation due to ill practices.

About the Book

Because this book covers some higher initiations in the Yogic spiritual path, this book will be different from most of the other books available to date. Yes, these will be all the things you already know, but you need to learn how to apply them. All the spiritual theories were there, but the practical activations were available only to a few. This is one of those books that make these profound initiations practically available in the most refined form to everyone.

Spiritual Fragmentation

SPIRITUAL FRAGMENTATION IS A RARELY discussed concept among yogis and practitioners. It also means spiritual madness or dysfunctional spirituality. Fragmentation begins the moment someone is taught that there is a higher world, power, consciousness, or purpose, and the world is lowly, evil, unconscious or animal-like. The perception of such beliefs creates two states in a person; one experiences the mundane life as unacceptable, and the other projects a heavenly life as a great achievement. The rejection towards practical life and the human self slowly takes the form of fragmented states. It soon starts manifesting as spiritual experiences of higher dimensions or realizations. While in reality, these were two different fragments of inner resources created over long years of mental projections.

Spiritual practitioners with such perceptions are always in search of a higher world, purpose, and life path. While there is nothing wrong with a perception of higher qualities, the harm is caused by self-rejection towards the practical life and the human self. No projected higher force is greater than the human self projecting it. The spiritual teachings must become clear in these aspects. Nowhere is it taught that all spiritual beliefs and experiences are created in self and have nothing to do with the higher world. By the time people come to face reality, it becomes too late. After decades of contemplating on a higher force, when someone realizes that the higher force is a projection of themselves, it would cause insanity. This is where the subconscious defence system hides it as something to avoid or fear. And this is how evil is born of the same reflection as the divine. It is there to protect reality and, ultimately, the creator from fragmentation.

But, this does not save the practical life of a person. The practical reality is said to be harsh because the feedback to dysfunctional behaviours and beliefs is never gentle. It would stand in the face until there is no option but to accept.

A practical explanation

Let us go into a practical perception of the entire experience.

A person in his/her teenage lives a gentle, normal life when motivated to have a great purpose in life. The great purpose could be anything. Now, what about the day-to-day life purpose? Practical life!

Because there is a great purpose that creates a sense of adventure and greatness, it makes one feel good. Still, in the infant projected state, the mind has experienced a state change that is much more desirable than daily life. How would that affect the connection with everyday life?

Of course, the person dreams more often of what feels better!!!

This is the first sign of state dissociation and dysfunction in practical life.

Depending on the intensity and time a person is living in the higher state, the presence in practical life will be affected. As people begin spiritual work, the intensity of experience peaks and most people tend to live in that state for years. What is expressed as an ungrounded state is another word for dissociation. In the dissociated state, it becomes altogether impossible for the person to do daily work or things that are in rejected mode. This creates a fall in every aspect of life as dysfunctional states and behaviours create chaos at work, in relationships, and in the family. And this is only realized by those around the practitioner, not the self.

Everything that forces the person to realize reality soon becomes a pain for the person. All of it is tagged undesirable, evil, negative energy, or whatever personalized metaphors have been taught. The problem is the fragmented state does not take care of your material needs. It is only one part of your emotional needs. The practical reality sooner or later will reveal that Happiness is a mundane thing, and you will not find it in higher dimensions.

This fragmented style of living takes a toll on the family, relationships, social life, and business. Most times, the damage is irreparable.

The antidote

Technically there is no recovery from this state after a decade or two of practicing dissociation. Life situations become so fixed over the years that only a few can reverse them. And none of the spiritual teachers and healers ever point it out at the very beginning.

Normally, this learning surfaces at its full force during the final spiritual initiation when the opposites begin to unify, and the field of unity is realized as the Non-Duality initiation. The test is caused by the practical reality and rational experiences vs what has been carried, projected and lived for years. Due to the spiritual state at the high, the mind tests and doubts every single thing and discards anything that does not serve a meaning. This is shock therapy for Spiritual Madness.

Spiritual Depression and Apathy

Some dedicated spiritual practitioners need to realize that their discipline has fallen into the trap of apathy. The person facing it is hardly aware of the situation and the reasons for spiritual apathy. This causes mental agony that is very different from depression to ordinary people. The emotions are similar to loss, separation, or major setbacks in life, but the structure of the situation is altogether different. The effect is soon realized in personal and practical life. Although it is possible to avoid this situation, people may suffer for years once in the trap.

The reason for the situation is the practice of non-attachment and disconnect from material pleasures. The letting-go process in the spiritual path is created to reach the non-duality state by dissolving the ego/personality. Because the human personality has a need for attachment to exist and function, the spiritual discipline creates an abrupt change in the entire structure. The problem is happiness is a mundane thing and is created by interaction in the physical world. The spiritual practice takes away a lot of things the person once enjoyed. This triggers state of self-denial and suppression, also causing the experience of loss. Any further practice in it would cause the mind to become apathetic in order to avoid suffering. The inner mind is no more mature than a three-year-old child. So, if you deny candy to a child, he solely desires, soon you will see the child acting cold.

In the early stages, this state feels like an achievement of non-attachment, but as soon as you call this child for action, you will get the same cold response. You have hurt the child and should not expect cooperation hereafter. This is how spiritual apathy is borne, and the seperative state is held as the agony of denial. Most practitioners would end up in this trap, which is mostly the end of spiritual growth and also harms other aspects of life.

The scene of anxiety and panic attacks is somewhat rare in most practitioners. But if the non-attachment practice of letting go is practiced to its limits, the mind soon loses all reasons to exist. It will be a state of utter hopelessness and not having any reason to exist. This creates a state of losing self or dissolving, which triggers anxiety and panic attacks.

The mind exists in great integration with the body, and the dissolving of the mind also affects psychological states of the body. For example, a person's muscular strength depends on mental states because the mind experiences itself in connection to muscles. But when the dissolving process begins, most of this connection is lost, creating the odd experiences of kundalini convulsions in the body. The body mass, strength, and other physiological features changes after such spiritual experiences. And it is rare to see someone developing super strength: rather, damage is more prominent in the entire body. Because this damage is not on a physical or psychological level, the repair process may take years as the mind restructures and anchors back in the body.

The situation might be pretty blissful if the practitioner is in a spiritual surrounding. The same would be chaotic in the life of ordinary people. Such people, though highly wise and vibrant end up being dysfunctional in daily life and work. It is quite impossible for them to do even the tiniest of daily work during the peak stages. And if proper care is not taken, the suffering and agony may take a toll.

This is where discipline plays its role. The mind may not exist, but the teachings, practice, and spiritual discipline will take over the void for the time the rebirth process continues.

If activated through such a process without proper discipline, a person living an everyday life may find self in odd states as a sudden change in emotional and mental states cause confusion and disconnect. It takes some time to tune up in the new field. A full awakening in such an environment might look like a psychosis episode or mental breakdown.

The current world scenario

The above scenario was true until the 90s because the teachings were only imparted to a few chosen disciples. This day, a large population is in practice by choice or by situation. The spiritual abilities of a guru have reached out to so many through reiki like healing modalities that there was a mass explosion of spiritual practitioners and teachers in just a decade. The internet has brought the rarest spiritual knowledge from the Himalayas to everyone on their mobile screens. And so, with it, the disciplines and belief systems have evolved into mass-level variations.

People are practicing all sort of modalities and expanding their consciousness in all possible ways. So with it, new difficulties too showed up. One of the major ones is the fragmented spiritual teachings, where the self is not the source of personal experiences. The dark and evil concepts, too, fall under this category.

Now, there is nothing wrong with any philosophy and practice as long as it gives the right results. The mass explosion of gurus has also brought to the notice that an outer guru is not always necessary. The path is to find the inner one.

Some paths may have harsh experiences, and some go with ease, but each one has its learning and growth.

The Field optimization

It seems the conscious energy field is making robust changes in the past few years. The earlier versions of spiritual activations could not be shared from a distance and used to take years to integrate. In current times the activations are shared beyond borders and through various mediums. The time it used to take for complete integration of any spiritual activation has reduced. And the severity of spiritual symptoms has been negated by recent teachers working to anchor spiritual energies and then sharing with all. Many people receiving these activations go through the transformation process with great ease. Also, there are the ones who choose the challenging process and later refine it further.

Dark Experiences

It is quite common to get into dark spiritual experiences during certain stages of spiritual practices. Most of these experiences are rooted in the call for help from your inner child that has been neglected and denied in the name of spiritual discipline. Other reasons for negative experiences are due to the dysfunctional spiritual teachings in culture. Most negative experiences dissolve as one becomes more receptive and attentive to self.

Some Clarifications

- The human mind has the ability to perceive and experience everything as one desires.

- Just because someone is experiencing something does not make it a practical reality.

- The perceptions generally dissolve as the subconscious desire or goal is reached.

- Ghosts, aliens, entities, and angels, good or evil, exist only in mind and are created in the space of personification. A disciplined tool created with personification could be realized in Bhakti Yoga.

- There are as many Gods as the number of human personifications.

- Metaphoric correlation is the secret ingredient of all spiritual responses. It could be used to create any form of spiritual healing system due to the placebo effect. It also stands true for the Nocebo effect. People make their own negative experiences with their own mental creations. The reason could be anything hidden from the conscious mind.

- Creating something in imagination and getting a response does not mean it will appear in physical reality. Expecting so creates the cognitive distortion of magical thinking. It is a sign that one lacks the needed skills to reach the goal.

- Nothing, practically nothing, has ever defied the laws of Physics, Chemistry, or even Biology. Psychology is the only flexible space but with lots of limitations. It is much more fruitful to align and work with the laws of practical reality than run in the magical beliefs.

- Supernatural powers never existed, nor will they ever will. Believing or needing one may have links to childhood bullying and abuse.

- Two people experiencing the same God experience them very differently based on their personal values.

- Bad or evil experiences are a sign of the internal defence system being triggered due to long-term stress. It means the system will not be able to stand anymore. It may also be a call for help at the onset of mental health issues. This space gets triggered during some spiritual techniques leading to distorted concepts.

- People who had spiritual experiences got them first in some extreme situations. There is a reason healthy people do not get them.

- A miracle is a result of a multistep process that the mind cannot comprehend.

- Once the mind has experienced something, it has all the needed resources to recreate it or even teach others to have a similar response.

- Spiritual energy is a response created with mental focus. Every piece of information and its metaphoric correlation will create a unique vibe.

- If you are not getting the desired result, you are missing some key points.

- If you are still reading, you are probably doing it too seriously. Do not take things that serious. A sign of transformation is a subtle sense of freedom in everything.

What makes one Unworthy

FOR OVER FIVE YEARS, I have tried writing this book innumerable times. For one reason or another, I was buzzed out and went mentally frozen. I have always believed that this discipline has to be practiced with purity in food and life habits. It was impossible to continue the spiritual cleansing to integrate the yogic activation with non-vegetarian food habits at home. I had the idea to drop this concept multiple times as pretty unique books are already complete.

What made me unworthy to write this book? My PI once said that it is impossible to write a single thing on these yogic kriyas unless there is permission from a higher authority. Now, where do I find the higher authorities?

The publication contract money has been borrowed from a few people and is going to waste. More of it, nothing in my career seems to be moving, unless I complete these tasks at hand. Neither can I force the process nor wait for it any further.

When I shifted to Chandigarh, I switched completely to vegetarian, never ate after 7:30 pm, and practiced yoga every day.

If yoga and vegetarian food were enough to hold this level of discipline, the book must have been released by now. There are still missing links even after a few thousand behavioral correction sessions.

Now, I was planning to leave Chandigarh for another city and get a teaching job. These days, I spend hours mostly in my room staring at my laptop screen, expecting the lines to flow. And then this coldness has taken over: No job, a career in total failure, no money, job offers worse than undergraduates, and this suppressed anxiety layered with disgust. Coldly watching the screen and doing nothing for hours and then for days, it was taking over my nerves. As I struck the coldness, a deep feeling of disconnect from the meaning of life surfaced. Apathy must be about ten of thousand layers deep to take so long to appear, even after years of emotional work. As the apathy meditation was shared with people, what showed up as a major reason of apathy was trauma indirectly linked to integrity.

Integrity is the most essential frequency that creates the soul or the attribute that structures the Personality (ID). Misalignment with this attribute makes one unworthy to receive, hold, or practice a high spiritual discipline. This level of spiritual activations might cause mental fragmentation if received by people lacking integrity, and even the wisest of the individual would not be able to defy this outcome.

Finally, when this chapter was written, it was almost a year of being vegetarian, but then during holidays, vegetarian food was discontinued. Even with non-vegetarian food intake, it is possible to practice this type of spiritual discipline, provided it aligns with your inner values. And with this realization, all strict rules so far has been lifted from this discipline. It does not matter what your habits and patterns are; if they are healthy and in integrity, you may practice this work.

Ultimately, this chapter gives a concrete meaning to spiritual purification. This technique may also be called the Kriya or Mudra of Integrity.

Though the simplification may have dimmed the charm of the discipline, it has the power to protect the practitioner from all possible corruptions and distortions in the spiritual world. And this attribute finally restores the soul body after a spiritual awakening and keeps one free of dark and fragmented spiritual journeys.

Nature of Personality

IN REFERENCE TO THE PERSONALITY model shown in the image: A State refers to a person's thoughts, feelings, emotions, behavior, and overall health. The most natural state is like a child at a very young age. The healthy state refers to the new forms learned and applied in the current environment, family, and social circle.

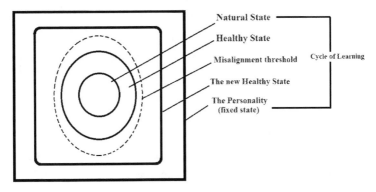

Structure of Personality

Misalignment begins with stress, pain, suffering, drama, disease, loss, or trauma. There is a threshold upto which misaligned states are naturally reversible in a short time or after an overnight sleep. But a continued misalignment creates and anchors new level of conditions that are not very natural to the person. Soon the person adapts to the new state that allows him to be functional in the environment. The personality, a structure formed of fixed states, is now an operating entity in the background and functions entirely from its pieces of information and learning. The learning cycle continues as new information layers are learned and anchored into the personality. This is the functional aspect of any person, and the personality may have hundreds of layers and cycles of formations.

Returning to Natural State

It is not in human instincts to stay far from our natural state. The personality keeps striving to return to its natural state at any given point in time. This is the core process all through life. When a learning process completes, we return to our closest, most natural state, integrating all lessons. Then we begin a new cycle. Being stuck in environments that misalign us from the natural state creates chaos. The personality continues to seek the path to return to its natural state.

The New Paths

It is natural for the personality to flow back to its original state. If it does not happen for a reason, the personality begins to function from the new layer while always looking for a way to return to its original state. This is the phenomenon of a call for help or a search for healing.

The personality may choose multiple other measures from the collection of available information. It cannot differentiate between healthy and unhealthy choices. But the options in the process decide the outcomes. Some may choose healthy patterns like exercise, creativity, art, or hobby. At the same time, there are those who choose addictions, indulgence, fights, and antisocial behaviors. The core nature is still to find that natural state and feel at home.

Depending on the available information and the environment (family, friends, social circle, education, media), the personality may choose anything that sounds appealing and effective. The choices themselves start a new cycle of learning. Most healthy behaviors assist in realigning with the Natural state depending on the amount of misalignment, the magnitude, and the length of the experience. In contrast, unhealthy behaviors create a short relief and add new layers of misalignment. Over time, these layers of consciousness become fixed and more petrified, making it impossible to reverse.

The Path of Healing

Healing is about releasing the misaligned states, integrating the reasons for misalignment, and realigning back with the natural state. While the memories and experiences cannot be erased: the emotions, feelings, and relative choices may be aligned. The healing is primarily natural for everyone. At times help from outside is required. Several modalities and therapies are available these days for people who seek help.

The Rebirth Process

The personality is only a projection of consciousness that is functional through the layers of the formation. It only exists as long as the material experiences and the need to function through these layers live. A major shift appears in consciousness when these layers and the reasons that hold on to these layers fall off. There is a sudden collapse in the entire personality structure and a total return to True nature. This is the process of Awakening or Enlightenment. It may also appear as spontaneous remission from overall issues in life.

The personality will cease to exist for some time, and then a new consciousness begins to structure; aware, refined, and radiant. The ability to connect with true nature allows the being to retune, refine and renew every moment. The experience also gifts a natural ability to step in and out of the layers as desired. This is where the personality is replaced by a Universal nature.

Seven Initiations

WHEN IT COMES TO NEW age spirituality, there are a few terminologies very closely used; Activation, Attunement, Initiation, and the Indian terms; Shaktipath and Diksha. To keep the subject free from confusion, each word is precisely defined. Other authors may or may not use these terms in similar references.

Activation is any kind of spiritual process, and it could be attunement, Shaktipath, or initiation. Attunement means connecting and tuning in to a different state or energy. It is a process of receiving spiritual energy from a teacher or a consciousness source. Sometimes the effect of the induced consciousness is temporary. Shaktipath and Dikkha/Diksha are Indian terminologies for attunement. Some also call it initiation. But for this subject, the term initiation is redefined.

Initiation is a very natural process. It is the integration of past experiences and life lessons. Spiritual initiations are nothing like attunements and cannot be received from a teacher or master. The outer teachings and attunements may help in the process, but the individual will be solely responsible for attaining progress. Initiations take years to complete and depend entirely on the realizations of the practitioner. Some spiritual systems identified the seven levels of initiations a practitioner goes through in life. The 7th initiation is said to be the completion, reaching the complete cycle of Soul liberation and attainment. Each initiation takes many years, and primarily 4th is the best achieved by most practitioners. In this work, initiation means both the beginning and the completion process. It represents completion because all the lessons and programs one has carried for years will integrate and reach completion. And it means a new beginning because, after the integration, the individual is no more the same.

The Seven Chakras and Initiations

The initiates in any yogic or spiritual system go through 7 levels of natural initiations over many years of practice. Depending on the ability to learn and integrate the life lessons, these initiations take a few years to decades to complete. The kundalini practice has two cycles of 7 years, i.e., it takes 14 years to complete the seven initiations. Some teachers explain it as the activation of the seven chakras and the awakening of the kundalini.

Each initiation goes through a process of information flow, learning, changes, and tests in a natural flow of life. Every initiation works in multiple planes and levels, out of which some are known or experienced by the initiate as changes in life situations, while others stay at the subtle level. The intensive process begins only for those who choose to take the path of intense practice. For others, it remains a subtle learning process in day-to-day life lessons and experiences.

The seven levels are explained as under:

1: Responsibility for Body and Health

This phase goes through education in body care and health. Sometimes it begins with health issues and self management lessons. It may take 2-3 years to complete this initiation. It has to do with root chakra attributes and discipline.

2: Responsibility of Passion

This phase goes through seeking your likings, passions, and a promising career. One may try multiple things to experience an expansion.

3: Responsibility of Self Power

Being able to handle self-power is the third major initiation. Practitioners may go through times of personal attack, criticism, and abuse or bullying from others. Being able to manage the states and master the emotions is a major lesson.

4: Developing self Love

This is a rough phase as the initiate is moved away from everything that brings love, affection, and connection. Everything one is attached to falls apart. This is a phase of solitude and emotional longing. Developing the inner sense of serenity and self-love without attention from others is a key learning. One turns out to be more compassionate and unconditional in this initiation. A stuck process may also cause modes of apathy for some time.

5: Healing the Past scars

While the past four initiations sound not much, in practical reality, the mind experiences them in a painful way. Remember, the entire drama and suffering is in the mind. But again, unless the conditions are fulfilled, the mind does not let go easily, and the past keeps repeating unless one choose to heal. Most people at this point seek help or learn the ways to heal themselves. Some even develop healing abilities as the need shows up. This phase goes through lots of inner work and healing, integrating the past lessons in a refined way. The initiate also may turn to work with others. Generally, this, too, is a reflection of inner work.

6: Final Test

Actual awakening or enlightenment is at the 6th initiation. It is more of a test of the past five initiations and the final integration of all soul lessons. Not an easy phase as unintegrated learnings, fears, unhealthy states, experiences, and emotions begin to surface. This is a phase where the personality dissolves or the soul body layer is removed, and the Universal self begins to take over. The person changes in every aspect of life as a radiant being. But before the light, there is the darkness and thunder, the Test of Non-Duality.

7: Completion

All the lessons as a human transform into energy and realign in the spiritual template from where the soul descended. The person becomes a source of never-ending wisdom and infinite spiritual consciousness.

The Ascended Chakra system

It is not essential to know the technical information about chakras and their process of integrating the initiations. The role of a practitioner is to flow with life lessons. Sometimes, working with the seven chakra system is helpful when stuck in a particular situation, but to depend entirely on chakras as the ultimate process may be misleading. Chakras were created as tools of refinement in consciousness; they are not the ultimate goal.

This further information is shared to offer a clear vision of the upcoming changes in consciousness and the chakra system.

The lessons in seven chakras

During the process of chakra transformation, the lessons and attributes in the seven chakras amplify to their full activity. It may take days to weeks for a chakra to cleanse and retune. Even complete kundalini activation, in one instance, stays focused on one chakra at a time before moving to the one above. Warming and electric flushes are common during the process. Along with it, the primary learning, emotions, and life experiences related to the chakra will surface and keep repeating until it harmonize and integrates. Episodes of emotions, memories, anger, irritation, headache, stomach issues, fear, etc., keeps showing up and releasing. At times flushes of golden light may seem to flow in the chakras. This phase may continue for few weeks, and the completion is marked with intense peace and bliss: a feeling of homecoming, joy, bliss, and groundedness. This is the completion of your Ascension and 5th Initiation. One may also receive a lot of synchronicity and messages about the completion process.

All major and subtle learnings from the seven chakras will first complete and integrate. Then the chakras begin to shift the energies to higher levels downloading and activating new layers of the chakra system that aligns with the seven major chakras. This will be a whole new level of energies, abilities, and learnings aligning with the person. Completion of the 5th initiation usually leaves the chakras changed to golden color.

For years, the chakra system might stay golden, and the practitioner may or may not choose to serve with spiritual skills. During the seventh initiation, the chakra may change colors to various combinations. The meanings of these new colors are unknown for now.

The Test of Non-Duality

IT IS DURING THE SIXTH initiation a practitioner comes across the stage what may be named the Test of Non-Duality. Similar to a learning process, the point of threshold whereby it is decided if one will continue or fall back. It is rare to find yogis who have been through the Test and ascended to self-realization.

Very little information is available on this topic among practitioners. All that has been propagated is about the wonders of the spiritual life. The dark side is kept hidden or unknown to many. Once in a while people at the peak of their seeking end up in areas that are better kept undiscovered. It is when they are at the height of their spiritual luxury the darkness appears: born in the light they have been using for years. This darkness is the result of their lightwork and cannot be cleared or destroyed by the spiritual gifts they have. This is where the Test begins.

How and when this level gets triggered is unknown. Stories of people who had these experiences are removed from this book. The reason is, such stories create induction in anyone reading or listening to it, producing a spontaneous meta-response. This induction effect has been observed multiple times and could be avoided if the stories are not taken that seriously. But people experiencing them project their illusions with such level of assurance that it gets imprinted to anyone.

Again, how a yogi or practitioner experiences this stage is entirely based on their practice and perception of the process. There is no clear definition or known process. Also, there is no way to find out what forces decide the Test and the outcome. What we know is that a person goes through intense overwhelming experiences during this phase.

Some explain it as an intense form of kundalini experience that continues for weeks. The chakra cleansing symptoms are much stronger than usually experienced. The healing system the person has been a master for years stops working for them. This follows a series of experiences that connects with their darkest insecurities and fears. Things stop making any sense, and there is a repeating cycle of past experiences at full intensity. At times the person might seem disconnected from reality or partly insane.

The experiences depend on personal beliefs and inner values. It is like a play at its most intense that a person has been living all his/her life. There will be a point of final choice somewhere, and things will slowly go normal. But there is no way to stop it, and there is no way to fail it. The process keeps repeating until it has reached the point of choice; right or wrong is unknown or indefinable. People or healers who have tried to intrude in the process by any means too get thrown up in an overwhelming experience. At times this energy is transferable and gets activated to anyone connecting with the knowledge or experiences of the initiate. As a safety measure, this is kept secret by most spiritual groups.

Most practitioners leave the spiritual path after this point as they realize the source of their spiritual essence and the meaninglessness in it. All the spiritual teachings and philosophies feel totally empty after that. At the spiritual level, the conscious field breaks the limited body of the soul and expands multi-dimensionally. This is where the highest discipline is needed, at the same time, there must be the readiness to savor the madness. There is no better term for this stage, with the flow of bliss at its peak that would engulf anyone interacting with the practitioner.

Religion, philosophies, spirituality, god, and any other concept become meaningless as the person realizes the supreme madness as the creator. This Being becomes the source of all and certainly cannot make sense in following anything created by self.

It takes a few years before the individual again begins to structure the ID, as will be visible by practical life activities. The Test has been completed, and the new being has been in the restructuring process. Most of this experience is forgotten, and the past seems non-existent. However, the creative gifts continue to manifest at times needed.

The Universal Circuit

THIS BOOK SHARES A 21 days meditation practice with a yogic mudra or hand posture. This technique of yoga has been practiced for thousands of years in India. The uniqueness of this work relies on the activation and the mudra practiced in the entire process. The mudra or the specific hand position acts as the switch to connect the circuit of higher consciousness through all dimensions of consciousness. The intensity and depth of the process depend on the time a person holds the mudra.

The concept was inspired by the technique of anchoring in NLP, the use of symbols in reiki, the mudra practice in yoga, and certain designs in Indian temples. A specific design from Shiva temples acts as the key activation or Shaktipath to this entire work. The early forms of this technique were directly taught by spiritual teachers with a mantra. In this work, the mantra has been replaced with a design to designate the direction and flow of the energy. The design also designates the trinity gods of creation.

21 days of purification

The main goal of this work was to introduce the reader to an effective tool that could be practiced and empowered in any environment. At the same time, the 21 days of practice lead to the development of a powerful transformational consciousness that would transmute any energy that the practitioner interacts with thereafter.

The practice aims to create, refine, and align to a set of pure values. The continued practice empowers the inner state and also refines the consciousness. After 21 days, environmental influence is allowed in this space, creating a flow of all types of new information. The effect is a powerful induction, purging, and refinement of any information.

The long-term effect is Dynamic Transformation in all aspects of life.

The concept of Purification

There is lack of a clear definition in the concept of spiritual purification. It is believed that there is impurity, negative energy, or karma that needs to be cleared. In a way these are metaphoric correlations to the desired goal. A clear definition and well-desired representation would help in reaching the goals with ease.

The Nature of personality model represents the cycle of life experiences and the development of the personality. The natural state would be the child aspect, untainted by life experiences but lacking needed maturity. The healthy state is where a person starts to function after a set of life experiences (both good and bad). This layer is formed with a set of beliefs, emotions, philosophies, and a collection of inner triggers. Any type of experience in life that crosses the threshold might not allow the person to shift back to normal or healthy space. These are generally the harsh lessons in life. But the mind learns to live in the new space and soon structures accordingly. This is where the person learns to handle both good and bad events, and emotions. It is a long-term negativity that generally leaves a person distorted: as it takes longer to settle into a new healthy space.

This is generally the making process of human personality. The layers were formed of information perceived or created in the mind, life experiences, and personal choices. In general expression, there is both good and bad information stored. A more technical term for bad would be Dysfunctional or Distorted, as they do not lead the person to a healthy goal or might even mislead.

What purification or spiritual purging would mean in a psychological setup would be applying a set of Positive Values to each layer of consciousness and aligning the information already stored inside. Anything misaligned with the set of values would be redefined in the scale of healthy values. It sounds easy in technical terms but is rarely possible without a set of effective Neurolinguistic tools. These layers form the experience of self, and it is rarely in a person's awareness to access these layers and make changes.

The technique to be profoundly effective, needs proper personal definitions of the process, the goal, a roadmap, and dedicated practice to empower the effects. Also, it is advised to self-clarify any doubts or misleading beliefs in the preparation stage itself.

This book has been written at its best to provide the complete structure of the process.

Prepare for the Initiation

PREPARATION FOR A SPIRITUAL ACTIVATION goes through multiple stages. Some yogic systems have rigorous initiation processes, while some have moderate rules. When it comes to natural initiations, the flow is governed mainly by personal beliefs and values. In this technique, the initiation and the later practice govern all needful changes in the consciousness. It would be helpful to begin the process with some discipline. There are some basic rules one must follow during and after initiation and the course of practice. This allows ease in opening up, receiving the flow, and maintaining the path of learning, at the same time avoiding major hurdles created by personal distortions.

Aspiration

The first and foremost point of initiation is the aspiration to realize the self. There is no point in participating in disciplines that do not align with personal aspirations. Also, it is against spiritual laws to activate people into any yogic discipline without their consent and full participation. Also, it would not be a fruitful path taken for the sake of learning yogic techniques or developing yogic powers. Healing and spiritual skills develop during the practices, but the effects are short-lived and may not produce concrete, practical results. The goal of a discipline must be free from aspirations of gaining any spiritual powers.

This level of the spiritual system is also not for a professional career in healing and coaching. Those abilities anchor at the fifth initiation but may get dissolved or get dysfunctional at the sixth. Participation to reach success in life may or may not bring effective results. Aspiration to realize the true self is the only way the aspirant reaches a path of learning and growth beyond imagination and conscious thinking.

Spiritual aspiration is natural to many or induced by life circumstances as a need to know the self. Some masters also described that spiritual learning and aspirations transcend all realities and get passed down from earlier lifetimes. The aspiration itself begins the process and flow of universal energies. It allows you to work through all tests and hurdles.

It is not hard to discern between spiritual aspirations and aspiring for spiritual path for material fulfillment. The second path ends up somewhere as soon as the mind receives the material aspects.

Ask yourself why you would like to take this path and where you would like to be. Reflect on the answers. There is no right and wrong in whatever the answer is. Accept and work with it.

Purification

Some people consciously choose purification, while many go through it unknowingly. It is important that the initiate goes through the purification physically, mentally, emotionally, and spiritually before any further process begins. As the initiations start, every aspect of life amplifies and surfaces. With unhealthy behaviors and habits, issues would arise sooner or later.

Discipline

Most of the problems in the new age spirituality are rooted in the lack of discipline. People are receiving initiations before proper inner work and purifications, which amplify the many layers of unhealthy consciousness. This is well reflected in the teachings and theories of new-age spirituality. The struggle and conflicts of the initiates are projected into the collective consciousness amplifying the spiritual combat people believe they are a part of. It takes a long time for most to realize the experiences are another paradigm play entirely controlled by old programs they thought no more existed. Consciousness has so many layers and sub-layers that it cannot be wholly explained in 12D theories.

Again pointing out the truth that there is no right or wrong. It is just about becoming aware and then becoming more aware: refining the realizations further every time.

Taking Initiations

Taking initiations isn't in the control of the personality. The only thing in control is the choice to take the spiritual path. Initiations naturally happen after a certain phase of spiritual work and maturation. All an initiate is needed to do is continue the practice and flow with the learning.

Ordinary people, too, go through these initiations but at a very slow pace that, at times, there is no realization of it. It all seems like the flow of life and circumstances.

For a dedicated yogi, there are times of sudden shift with major surfacing and later a time of ecstasy and bliss. This process begins after many years in practice. Usually, this is the most natural type of initiation people go through. The level of awareness and perception is highly raised at this time.

There is another source of spiritual initiation. Some people go through natural initiations at sacred sites. This is due to the high energy vortexes that allow fast processing of information and integration, completing the initiation. But this happens only when the initiate is ready from within.

The Test of Non-Duality

There is a third way to it, like the commoner, by working with the learnings offered in daily life, which at a subtle level is the process of initiation. A focused working creates a faster pace of integration and upgrade to the successive initiations. While this level of awareness is developed only by higher initiates, it could be learned from them.

The Activation

VARIOUS YOGIC SYSTEMS USE MANTRAS for spiritual activations. Reiki, specifically uses Japanese symbols for attunements. The concept of spiritual symbols in India includes the inscriptions in ancient temples. It is said that symbols are the keys to activating spiritual consciousness. The symbols are specifically used to anchor and store spiritual activations for later generations. A vast collection of such inscriptions can be found in Indian temples. The activation in this book has been inspired by one such symbol mostly found in Shiva temples. It is more of a simplified geometry to use in the activation.

The Sacred symbol holds all the needed energy and information to activate the process. In the process of spiritual awakening, a practitioner comes across hundreds of such geometrical designs. It is said that the sacred geometries are followed by everything in this Universe. Multiple yogic systems work with sacred geometries defined with yoga postures to align with the universal consciousness. These sacred symbols hold multidimensional programs and energies beyond our ability to interpret. The knowledge of these geometries and their possible meaning was most probably known by Indian Yogis. Hence, these geometries are spread across sacred places and temples. The Yogis realized the capacity of the human brain and the nature of the spiritual energy field. The deep understanding that these sacred symbols could hold a tremendous amount of information that could be ingrained and activated later on could be transformational. The most effective way to connect with any sacred geometry is through direct interaction, touch, feel, and sight. But they don't activate for everyone. There is a certain level of spiritual field needed for the person to activate the keys. Once that happens, the symbol itself will reveal everything. These multidimensional keys are around all the time, and people are in no way aware of their presence and energetic interactions as they are inactive or locked without the presence of a vibrational field. They need activation before all the information and energy flow is received.

The activation is very specific and has to be done on the proper site covering the right chakras. There is no second activation for this type of spiritual activation neither is there a reversal process. The energy activation could be as intense as fully active kundalini energy and might not be a smooth experience with some practitioners.

How to Activate?

The activation design has been shown in the later images. The design covers the three lower chakras; root, sacral, and solar plexus. The energy spinning begins at these chakras as the design is activated. After that, during the practice, the energy moves to higher chakras in 21 days process. This is a self-attunement, and the readers must perform the process on themselves. After the practice is complete, the same process could be used to activate others.

Use your imagination to activate the design. Sit on the ground, close your eyes and meditate. Imagine you leave your seat and walk to the back side of your body. See your spine and back. Focus your mind on the three lower chakras. Use your index and middle finger together and draw like the middle finger is the tip of a paintbrush (in your imagination). Draw the symbol in three steps; the line, an anticlockwise circle on the solar plexus, and then the triangle, the base of which passes the root chakra. This is the complete activation. Continue to meditate for 15-20 minutes and then take a nap.

When you wake up from the sleep meditation, remember to drink lots of water. Spend the day relaxing. You may also practice writing your session experiences for future review.

To activate this session for someone else, use the same technique of activation. The session could be activated both on a person in the same room or remotely. This information is for practitioners. But if you wish to educate someone in this process, let them read and work with the book first.

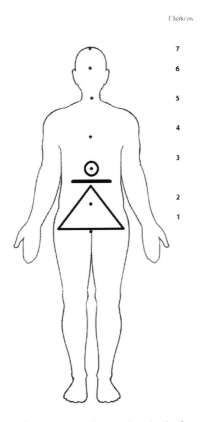

Sacred Design on lower back chakras

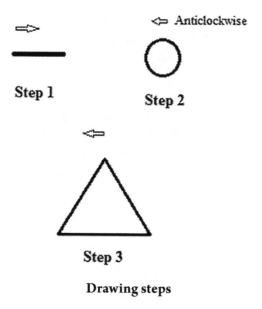

Drawing steps

The Practice

THE EARLIER CHAPTER SHARED THE activation process, and now it is time for practice. The spiritual circuit locked in the seven chakras system has been activated, and the key switch is in your palms. Holding the specific mudra (hand posture) during yoga or meditation completes the circuit and creates an intense flow of spiritual energy in the body and the field. The otherwise incomplete circuit is the reason for the lack of spiritual consciousness in daily life. This is the secret of Yogic practice, which took six years to decipher and make it into this chapter.

It is time for a dedicated practice for 21 days without any gap. The discipline of vegetarian food and no smoking or alcohol applies for as long as the practitioner chooses to work with this technique. The heightened states during the practice and intense flow of spiritual energy might cause severe issues if the body holds any impurity. It would be natural for all addictions and negative behavioural patterns to purge out during the practice.

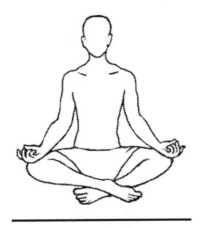

Sit on the Ground

The practice is simple. Sit on the ground or on your yoga mat, close your eyes, and keep your back straight, your palms resting on your knees, facing upward. Now hold the mudra. Gently touch the tip of your thumbs to the base of your ring finger. This is the purification mudra. The moment the mudra is made, the energetic flow begins. Meditate for 15-20 minutes. Practice for 21 days.

Multiple advanced mudras show up during these 21 days of practice, each of them holding a different consciousness.

Yogic practices become most effective when practiced daily and at a particular time. A fixed time is essential as the mind becomes programmed to participate daily, making it easier to focus. The second most important aspect of discipline is the dedicated timeline. Few people understand the meaning of having a timeline in practice. It is like goal setting or focusing on a particular outcome fixed to a specific date. Working with the timeline concept will reveal its effects later on. This is how you train to reach your spiritual goals.

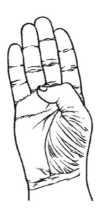

Hold the Mudra

Once a timeline is decided, all synchronicities and energies update the flow in alignment with the process decided. There will be very clear internal directions to reach the fulfillment of the process.

While it is impossible to align personal goals with the spiritual flow and trying to fix a timeline is like pushing yourself to a landmark with a deadline. This technique's purpose is to be conscious and stay open to the process. Also, it means only one layer of consciousness will be worked on at a time, and only after its complete refinement will the next level of work be chosen. When working with this tool, try not to expect too much in a very short time. Some Initiation processes may take months or years.

Over time the dedicated timeline process goes on auto mode as your natural spiritual initiations begin and goes along the entire life. This is where transformational living begins. Because everything you interact, experience, or participate in becomes integral to your learning and soul evolution.

Emotional Awareness

WE HUMANS USE EMOTIONS AS a radar for directions in life. We choose things as per our likes and dislikes. Something that feels bad is a no-entry signal. Things that feel good are the ones to whom we get attracted. This is where it is most crucial to have a clear awareness of emotions. The reason is this world functions on duality and is divided into good and bad projections. Things are both good and evil as per duality perceptions. At times the feel-good things may leave a person in long-term emotional pain. Emotional awareness is the ability to feel emotions deeply and be in tune with them all the time. Though forgotten, most past emotions are functional on the deeper layers of mind, and control all aspects of life.

The Source energy, through many dimensions, reaches the human spiritual field, the mental layers, the emotional, and finally, the physical body. Imbalanced and negative emotions block the flow of energies and connection to the spiritual self. While mental focus and thoughts create the Quantum field vibrations, emotions control the system. The vibes of a person are much more of the person's internal feelings. After some level of transformation, the emotional body begins to direct the flow of Universal energies.

Feeling your emotions and staying aware during this practice is one major step in transforming your emotional field.

The field of Emotions

Suppose a metaphoric scale is created to measure emotions. In that case, a person on a lower note will perceive everything from a perspective of survival mode and personal needs. The medium range brings a natural flow, and the person perceives more from balance and harmony. The higher scale brings in the path of Service and perception of the higher picture of life. The purpose of Ascension at human level is to learn and work with emotions. The higher dimensional work is for the higher aspects and not really in the choice of a person.

The lower the energy levels, the tougher to make corrections and heal. The problems stay longer and take long-term work before they resolve. Being on a higher scale allows flow, flexibility, and healthy emotions. The higher emotions and attributes are needed to correct the soul frequencies and move into higher consciousness. It is through life lessons and the complete integration of experiences we move into higher attributes. With each choice and experience (good or bad) there is a relative lesson. The completion of learning mostly allows a person to make more positive choices, and the relative frequency level is reached. This is frequency or soul-level corrections.

Everyone goes through the process of life-long learning and emotional tuning. The completion of a lesson and its integration could be truly named Initiation. Because once the learning completes, the person is no more the same and will not go back into old patterns and attributes. The purpose of spiritual work is not to manipulate this natural process. But to allow clear space for deep reflections and integrating the learnings. A healthier consciousness is developed through disciplined practice and it is applied in all aspects of life lessons. If a person has truly developed a clear space, then the application of the awareness to anything will create transformation in the life lessons, allowing a fast harmonization and integration of the lessons. This is one reason spirituality allows change in energy levels.

There are certain ways of being or keeping self on the Positive scale. This is possible for every common man. There is another way of raising the energy scale and that is by being associated with a person on a higher spiritual level, your spiritual teacher. It creates the induction effect.

The dark abyss

The dark abyss is a metaphoric expression of the negative emotional states beyond the conscious control of the mind. This is a multilayer formation, and the number of layers depends on individual factors like age, life experiences, behavior, etc. A person, over years of negative experiences, may fall really deep. The darkest layers lead to the most basic survival instincts, and the person does not really care for the outcomes in such a situation.

The slippery slope

Every being is born in the most natural happy space. Over years of life experiences and choices, new layers are formed that designate the person's personality. A person has control over life situations to a certain extent. Similarly, emotional states triggered by experiences are controlled by the mind. But when the threshold is crossed, there is no going back. This is called the slippery slope. Once the choice is made, the path ahead slips into the world's harsh realities, and there is no way back. The negative emotions and experiences become a fixed reality for the person.

This is called a slippery slope because every time the person tries to take control, there is a deeper fall.

People who easily reach their desires are less likely to fall into darker emotions and negative choices. As lack and unfulfilled states take over, the mind wanders closer to the dark abyss.

Healing

The early stages are easier to heal and recover from because there is a minor amount of negativity and damage. But the advanced layers may be a space of no return.

The path of healing goes through acceptance of emotional states in each layer and mentoring the person positively reach the core desires.

This is the challenging part. The mind might resist the new information of receiving the core desires.

The purging process

This yogic practice has a deep purging effect on the soul. Each layer surfaces, heals, and realigns in the most positive way available. The circumstances begin to shift as the polarities built over time get released.

This is the mentoring phase. The higher consciousness takes over the process assisting in healing and alignment.

Yogic Symptoms

ORIGINALLY, SPIRITUAL SYMPTOMS WERE NOT for dedicated yogis and spiritual practitioners. Most of these symptoms were known to people interacting with the yogis during their practice. Touching a yogi in meditation or Kriya naturally creates a flush of energy. The symptoms experienced were short-lived and quickly grounded. Mostly the energy flow is subtle and feels good to be around. But intense levels may cause severe symptoms like flu, body ache, nausea, deep trance, and emotional release.

These days the symptoms happen to everyone, especially if the surroundings are unhealthy. Once in a while, severe symptoms are generally caused due to sudden energy shifts. But if the symptoms are recurring, there is a lot of work to be done. Lack of discipline is the prime reason for these symptoms. The second most common reason for symptoms these days is induction due to reading about the symptoms. Hundreds of thousands of people have been facing planetary retrograde symptoms since they began following an astrologer or healer on social media. There is an apparent reason for these symptoms. People do not understand that they are being programmed to experience them. Also, spiritual seekers pick symptoms from other practitioners.

During the process of spiritual transformation, the layers of consciousness begin to open up, surfacing all old emotions and experiences. These states show symptoms, and the severity depends on a person's emotional history. As the layers open up, the consciousness shifts to its most natural state, causing a collapse in the layers of experiences that matured over time. This sudden collapse causes the flush of emotions, feelings, and memories through the body and mind, causing release symptoms. Some layers have intense pain associated with them. Clearing these layers may cause emotional and physical pain.

This is interesting to know that all these layers have a significant structure of pain, suffering, and fear programs, that were unknowingly picked from the surroundings. There is so much suffering that it takes years to clear it from the mind and body. Though the technique may have the effect of thousands of deep cleansing meditations, it took much more inner work before it could be shared. Anyone interested in teaching this technique must be well aware that it needs quite a time of dedicated practice before one could be genuinely ready to channel it to others. Otherwise, it would cause forceful cleansing of traumatic layers in consciousness, creating all types of symptoms.

Resistance and Attachment

The structure of personality is formed of layers of experiences and memories. It is natural that the release and clearing of these layers create a state of losing self. This triggers resistance to the process and limits the possibility of release. The personality shows states of panic as it may seem to be dying or reaching a non-existent state. It is normal for the personality to create new states and imaginations that would slow down the process for some time. These responses create all types of otherworldly experiences as a projection of the dissolving personality. Shedding of the old self may create insecurities, fear, and panic perceptions. This phase is experienced as both intense panic and fear, later shifting into total bliss. Such experiences take a peak during kundalini awakening and then show up at times as certain layers fall off.

Self care during Yogic symptoms

There is no proven way to avoid the yogic symptoms altogether. Though accepting the process creates an ease in the flow. It is essential that the practitioner stays calm and composed, irrespective of the inner turmoil. Staying away from crowds and troublesome people is suggested, as these are the sources of triggers. For unknown reasons, people too can sense the changes happening in a practitioner and generally are attracted to them, triggering specific emotional events. Out of all, the most important part is never to share spiritual experiences with others during the wave of changes, especially not with the non-practitioners. The inner changes and experiences might not make any meaning for others and show up as gibberish beliefs. At times these experiences also induce the listeners and create all types of odd experiences triggering fear in their minds. This is because spiritual experiences carry the field of energy and get transmitted with words. Although there would be immense changes happening within, it is not the refined form of wisdom to be shared. It takes some time after the integration for the refined information to express.

During the moments of silence, the primary lessons in life show up and integrate. Once that happens, the symptoms ease. During advanced spiritual work, a practitioner must work through core values related to life experiences. The overwhelming moments are the points of resistance, after which it shifts into harmony. In this phase, the body and mind are in a delicate flow and need proper care. There would be a continuous flow of information as old programs surface and retune. Misaligned and conflicting information from the outer world may cause chaotic states. Choices that raise the alarm may trigger inner conflicts.

The mind is in the phase of testing and will ceaselessly work to reach the goals by reviewing and retuning everything. At times the perception of the world might seem like an illusion, and then the idea of illusion itself might not make any meaning. The third eye experience creates experiences of heightened senses. This triggers experiences of cognitive distortions and magical experiences. Soon the mind realizes the power to choose the perception of everything and its balance with practical reality. People with spiritual faiths get supernatural experiences but soon realize how their own mind is playing it out. These events, too, connect with the symptoms one experiences in this phase.

It is said that the karmic cycle repeats itself and then finally gets released during the sixth initiation. The mind experiences everything as a reflection of self and clearly becomes aware of the results personal choices create. The cycle of karma speeds up at this time and almost instantaneously reciprocates any action.

Then, there is the need for proper rest that the body has been denied in a busy life. The heightened awareness also makes the body tired and creates a need to rest more than usual. The weariness is a sign that the body has not rested well in the past. The stress from the body and mind begins to surface as symptoms and dissolve after proper sleep. The yogi has to retune to a new schedule and life habits that are more appropriate to the current level of consciousness. It is beneficial to honor the body needs and rest as much as needed.

This is also the best time to develop healthy boundaries as the new set of programs reach the inner mind easily and manifest to their full potential. Healthy boundaries save a person from getting intoxicated by others around. Even if not by personal choice, the practitioner would suffer symptoms triggered by toxic traits from others.

Meditation and a dedicated practice align and harmonize the process and are a few ways to avoid any symptoms. Also, this daily dedicated time is the best inner space to be for people living in populated cities. The stored misaligned emotions and mental programs are subconsciously picked from people around. So a place where people are angry and frustrated about any situation will only trigger such emotions. This continuous bombardment of negative emotions will only taint the perception of life. A daily cleansing meditation is a way to maintain peace and serenity.

Food and Body needs

Being gentle to your own body is important when one takes the path of yogic discipline. Going through very strict diets and fasting practices least help through the transformation process if the body is not ready to take the shift. Tap into the wisdom of your body, connect, feel, and work accordingly. Actions and practices against your body will only hinder and blocks the flow.

The higher initiations are times of intense change in the body and field. The body changes in ways unknown on the surface in order to hold the universal energies. At this time, the body's needs may change all of abruptly. The old food habits may not be enough to nurture the body in this process.

Most times, the upcoming initiations are signaled by an excessive craving for sweets or chocolates. Even if one is not on heavy physical work, this means the body needs high sugar during these transitions. Sometimes, the craving for food can not be identified with certain food. It makes a person overeat or consume unhealthy stuff. Generally, food is not enough to satisfy this inner craving. Meditation and self-healing may help the need for spiritual energy that feels like a food craving. Visualizing healing light on food and water before intake is a known technique that is most effective in this situation. Fruits that are high in antioxidants also help in soothing the symptoms and cravings.

Some things that helped people

People tend to experience cravings for food that cannot be satisfied just by eating. In such moments lemonade and orange juice has shown great soothing effects. Intake of peaches and prunes twice or thrice a week helps ease many symptoms related to cleansing as well as the food cravings. Salt baths has been another popular practice these days to clear the energies. Soaking your feet in luke-warm water with salt soothes the hyperactive nerves.

Most important of all, when nothing seems to make sense and odd experiences are taking over, do not indulge in anything and go for a good sleep. This one habit will solve almost all problems, and protect you from getting in odd situations that are later regretted.

Reasons of symptoms:

1. For daily practitioners there are minor or no symptoms.
2. Symptoms are strong for those who do not practice daily. This is because of collection of information and energy that needs integration causing symptoms.
3. Opening up inner layers cause flow of past memories and emotions triggering symptoms.
4. Insensitivity to self / body/ not enough rest is a major reason.
5. Energy downloads – trying to integrate.
6. Retuning in core programs cause collapse in the outer structure of emotions and experiences.
7. Aspects/ parts taking over or surfacing to heal.
8. Dissolving personality.
9. Resisting to the process.

SHU HA RI

SHU HA RI IS A Japanese term that closely defines the transformation process with this work. This definition will govern the readers in practice and later pass on this tool to others. There are three stages in the process of learning and transformation. SHU is when someone learns something from a teacher. This is the first learning phase. It must be learned and worked exactly the way it has been taught, as not following the original template may create learning gaps. Then this type of work has other issues; the mind reaching enhanced states of awareness may wander off into unnecessary discoveries and get the disciple distracted in a self-projected and totally unhealthy space. That is why spiritual teachings and initiations are shared with disciples directly under the surveillance of a Guru. Suppose the teacher identifies distortions in the consciousness of the student; in that case, those are corrected before the disciple is allowed to take any activations.

The first stage of receiving itself feels like an achievement as a flow of joy and bliss is experienced. This could be the first 21 days, the first week of practice, or years in practice. It all depends on the practitioners. And then the next stage takes over. At this time, the student no more feels aligned with what has been taught. It feels dull and dysfunctional. The student loses interest in the original teachings and begins to wander off. Most people stop in this phase. It is a time of self-doubt and hardships in practice. The teacher and original teachings will not be able to answer the conscious needs of the student. The seeking continues, but the practice fragments. Some time passes, and one fine night a new flow takes over. A transformed knowledge begins to flow that is unique and vibrant. It shows up with enhanced joy and bliss, rejuvenating everything. This is the final stage.

The new information flows from the most profound creativity and brings with it a sense of fulfillment and bliss. The student is no more dependent on an external source for directions. The inner guru, at this point, has taken charge and true realizations flow from within the student. This is where the discipline becomes truly aligned with the most authentic and divine self. The new knowledge flows like the notes of music, unhindered by the gaps of the material mind. The consciousness at this point has reached the realization of the Source.

The first 21 days of this practice may go through many cycles of such realization until everything is completely transformed and integrated. The practitioner will know the point of completion without any doubt. There will be a creation of new ideas and tools in this phase that will be most aligned with the practitioner. And these new tools born from the practice would be unique and new to this field of consciousness. It would be different from what has been taught, pure, and unified with the soul consciousness of the person. At this phase, the student becomes a new teacher. And this is the form that would be passed down to the next generation of students.

Other half of Spiritual Awakening

THE TEACHINGS ARE SO FOCUSED on reaching higher consciousness or a higher reality that very few realize it to be the only half aspect of spiritual awakening. There is a second half to the process. It might have been well ingrained in the minds of seekers that spiritual awakening is a challenging task, and not everyone reaches it. But the reality is, it is pretty simple and easy to reach. What might come as the difficult part is the second half of the process.

Kundalini energy has always been shown to awaken and move to higher chakras, but that is not the complete scenario. After a few weeks, as the energy transcends the higher chakras, it begins to descend back and is received by the seven chakras and later anchors back in the personality. Even if the kundalini experience may work only for a few weeks, the complete descent takes a few years. The human soul, which has been dissolved in the sixth initiation, begins to restore, and the personality takes up new behavioral traits refined with spiritual work. This phase after the dark night of soul is the cocoon formation and it is normal for the person to feel disconnected from everything. The consciousness is integrating all the knowledge that has been collected in earlier phase and is in the process of transformation. It may take some years before the cocoon is broken and the wings of freedom are ready for the first flight.

It takes anywhere from five to seven years for the transformed personality to restructure and start functioning. The inner work and discipline may continue forever.

Testimonials

The few participants who received this content had got them mixed with the earlier books. For this reason, hardly any testimonials were received for this book. Let the testimonials now show up in reviews. The readers are requested to share their thoughts after the completion of practice.

I remember one event with this 21 days practice that a lady wrote back in 2018. Because it is related to the discipline, I clearly remember it.

The lady received the mudra activation and had a very intense energy purge with a huge rush of emotions. It was hardly a week, and I received her message that it was getting too intense and overwhelming for her to continue the practice. Also, she happened to take some wine at a party and thereafter had the worst emotional state.

The message is clear. Discipline means discipline, no playing around.

It would be interesting to learn about the reader's experiences with this practice.

Check the new website www.beyondplacebo.in for online sessions and coaching workshops. A new form of transformational coaching is in the launch process.

Book Series

Beyond Placebo

Beyond Placebo is the first book in this series. It shares a unique concept of healing with simple words. The purpose of the healing codes shared was to prepare the spiritual seekers for upcoming transformations by releasing the layers of trauma and abuse. All four books in series are connected in the flow of spiritual learning and transformation.

'I AM' Experiments

The second book in the series shares the healing journey of the author. The stories and realizations imbibe a powerful vibe transforming the readers.

Test of Non-Duality

The third book in series covers the hardships spiritual seekers and yogis has to go through before they reach realizations. The author shares the concept of darkness born of spiritual light as the hidden ignorance spiritual practices carry. Then, a intensive purification technique has been shared that assists practitioners release all distortions in consciousness.

Book 4

This book shares cycle of ascension into 24 major activations with Quantum Codes. It completes the complete cycle of ascension/ purification and embodiment of the higher consciousness.

Crystals Series

Celestial crystals is a series in making that would share the energetic attunement to all known crystals on earth. The collection of healing crystals from around the world has been going for few years now. The project is in collaboration with a crystal collector. The first part of this series Celestial Crystals shares the connection to Meteorites and Tektites.